RYAN STONE

Behind the Diagnosis

Personal Accounts of Overcoming Colon Cancer

First edition

This book was professionally typeset on Reedsy. Find out more at reedsy.com

Contents

1

INTRODUCTION

A person may experience life-changing emotions such as astonishment, awe, and fear after learning they have cancer. The process of adjusting to a cancer diagnosis requires time and help from family members and medical experts. This chapter will discuss the diagnostic's shock and offer advice on surviving the initial stages of a colon cancer diagnosis.

How to Deal with a Cancer Diagnosis News:

When someone learns they have cancer, their life is irrevocably altered. When given a cancer diagnosis, many patients say they feel as though a freight train has run over them. Common responses to news are shock, disbelief, and denial. When you receive a cancer diagnosis, you could feel scared, anxious, and uncertain about the future. It's crucial to give yourself time to absorb your feelings as coping with the news of a cancer diagnosis is a process that requires time.

Talking to your loved ones is one of the most crucial things you can do when adjusting to a cancer diagnosis. During this trying time, your family and friends can offer emotional support and serve as a source of strength. It's crucial to ask questions of your medical staff regarding your diagnosis, available treatments, and prognosis. You can feel more in control and make decisions regarding your therapy if you are well-informed.

Getting Help from Family and Medical Personnel:
Although getting a cancer diagnosis can be a lonely process, you don't have to do it by yourself. When dealing with a cancer diagnosis, family members and medical professionals should be consulted for support. Your family members can offer you emotional support, assist you with daily duties, and go with you to appointments. Your healthcare team can give you medical assistance, respond to your inquiries, and put you in touch with further services.

It's crucial to keep in mind that by asking for assistance, you are not putting a burden on your loved ones. They want to be there for you during this trying time. Other options, such support groups or social workers, are available if you don't have family or friends close by. They can assist you get in touch with local resources and offer emotional support.

Recognizing the Value of Early Detection:
Treatment of colon cancer depends greatly on early detection. The likelihood of successful treatment and recovery increases with earlier cancer detection. For people over 50 or earlier for those with a family history of the disease, routine colon cancer screening is advised. Fecal occult blood tests, stool DNA tests,

colonoscopy, and other screening techniques are available.

It's crucial to go over screening options with your doctor and to adhere to the prescriptions given your age and risk factors. It's crucial to contact your doctor as soon as possible if you experience any symptoms or have any worries. Changes in bowel habits, abdominal pain, blood in the stool, or unexpected weight gain are all signs of colon cancer.

It might be upsetting and overwhelming to learn that you have cancer. It takes time, support, and knowledge to process the news of a cancer diagnosis. It's critical to ask for help from family members and medical professionals, to be aware of your diagnosis, available treatments, and prognosis. Following suggested screening recommendations and discussing any concerns or symptoms with your doctor are vital since early discovery is crucial in the treatment of colon cancer. Even though receiving a cancer diagnosis can be a drastically altering event, it's crucial to keep in mind that there is still hope and that many people can successfully treat and recover from colon cancer.

CHAPTER ONE

Treatment Options: Making Tough Decisions

T he sort of treatment the medical staff suggests for a patient who has been diagnosed with colon cancer will rely on a number of variables, including the cancer's stage, the patient's general health, and other personal concerns. Chemotherapy, radiation therapy, and surgery are the three basic methods of treating colon cancer, though often a mix of these methods is advised for the greatest results.

Chemotherapy: This medical procedure employs chemicals to destroy cancer cells. These medications can be administered intravenously or orally, and they circulate throughout the body to eradicate cancer cells that might have spread outside of the colon. Before or after surgery, chemotherapy can be used to reduce tumor size and eradicate any cancer cells that may still be present.

Chemotherapy may target cancer cells anywhere throughout the body, even those that may have moved to other organs, which is one of its main benefits. A reduced immune system, exhaustion, nausea, vomiting, and hair loss are a some of the adverse effects of chemotherapy. To manage these side effects and keep their general health during treatment, chemotherapy patients must work closely with their medical team.

Radiation therapy: Radiation therapy is a medical procedure that destroys cancer cells by exposing them to high-energy radiation. It is frequently combined with other therapies like chemotherapy or surgery. Radiation therapy can be applied both before and after surgery to reduce tumors and eliminate any cancer cells that may still be present.

Radiation therapy is a localized form of treatment, i.e., it only affects the parts of the body where cancer cells are located. This can lessen the chance that the healthy cells and tissues surrounding the malignancy will sustain damage. Radiation therapy, however, can also have negative side effects such weariness, skin irritability, and organ damage. To minimize these side effects and maintain their general health throughout treatment, patients who get radiation therapy will need to collaborate closely with their medical team.

Surgery: The main form of treatment for colon cancer is surgery, which entails the removal of the colon's malignant tissue. Surgery aims to eradicate all cancerous cells and stop the disease from spreading to other parts of the body. A partial colectomy (removal of a segment of the colon), a total colectomy (removal of the entire colon), or a proctocolectomy (removal of the colon and rectum) may be advised depending on the stage of the cancer.

Open surgery, laparoscopic surgery, and robotic surgery are all options for doing surgery. The size, location, and general health of the patient will all be taken into consideration before recommending a surgical procedure. Depending on the procedure, recovery times can vary, but patients must collaborate closely with their medical team to control pain, watch for problems, and gradually return to their regular activities.

The optimal course of action for treating colon cancer will depend on a number of individual circumstances, including the cancer's stage, the patient's general health, and personal preferences. The three basic treatment modalities are chemotherapy, radiation therapy, and surgery; occasionally, a combination of these modalities may be suggested. To understand the advantages and disadvantages of each treatment option, control any side effects, and participate actively in their treatment plan, patients should consult with their medical team frequently. Many colon cancer patients can experience a successful outcome and return to a healthy, happy life with prompt and suitable treatment.

Balancing the potential benefits and risks of each option

When a patient is told they have colon cancer, the medical staff will go over the various treatment choices and assist the patient in choosing the best course of action. When deciding on the appropriate course of action, it is crucial to thoroughly analyze the potential advantages and disadvantages of each treatment option.

Chemotherapy: One of the key advantages of chemotherapy is its ability to target cancer cells across the body. This is particularly useful if the cancer has spread outside the colon. To improve the likelihood of a positive outcome, chemotherapy can also be combined with other treatments, such as surgery. A reduced immune system, exhaustion, nausea, vomiting, and hair loss are a some of the adverse effects of chemotherapy. The medical staff will go over these possible dangers with the patient and offer assistance in managing any potential side effects.

Radiation therapy: To improve the likelihood of a favorable outcome, radiation therapy is sometimes combined with other therapies like chemotherapy or surgery. One of radiation therapy's advantages is its capacity to target cancer cells in a particular body region, which lowers the possibility of causing harm to healthy cells and tissues nearby. Radiation therapy, however, can also have negative side effects such weariness, skin irritability, and organ damage. The medical staff will go over these possible dangers with the patient and offer assistance in managing any potential side effects.

Operation: The main form of treatment for colon cancer is surgery, which entails the removal of the colon's malignant tissue. One of surgery's advantages is that it can eradicate all cancerous cells and stop the disease from spreading to other parts of the body. Surgery does, however, come with dangers, such as the potential for bleeding, infection, and harm to adjacent organs. The medical staff will go over these possible dangers with the patient and offer assistance in managing any potential side effects.

Patients should collaborate closely with their medical team to comprehend the options available and make an informed decision because weighing the possible benefits and dangers of each treatment option may be a challenging task. When recommending a course of therapy, the medical staff will consider the cancer's stage, the patient's general health, and personal preferences. To ensure that they are at ease with the chosen course of action, patients should express their concerns, look for second views, and participate actively in their treatment plan.

Patients should take additional aspects into account, such as their quality of life while undergoing therapy and their long-term prognosis, in addition to the potential advantages and hazards of each treatment option. For instance, while some patients may prioritize a treatment that delivers a greater quality of life while undergoing treatment, others may favor a treatment that offers a higher possibility of curing them. To make a choice that feels right to them, patients should explore these factors with their medical team and close family members.

In conclusion, it is crucial for patients with colon cancer to weigh the potential advantages and disadvantages of each treatment option when making a choice. In order to comprehend the options available, ask questions, and make an informed choice that takes into consideration their unique requirements and preferences, patients should collaborate closely with their medical team. Many colon cancer patients can experience a successful outcome and return to a healthy, happy life with prompt and suitable treatment.

Personal stories of individuals who chose different treatment paths

People with colon cancer can learn a lot about the various treatment options and their possible advantages and disadvantages by reading personal accounts. For those dealing with a cancer diagnosis, hearing from others who have gone through similar experiences can be a source of motivation and useful insights into the decision-making process. Here are some instances of personal accounts from people who selected various treatment trajectories:

Chemotherapy was suggested for Mary after her colon cancer was determined to be in stage 3 and she underwent surgery and chemotherapy. Because of the probable adverse effects, Mary was concerned about chemotherapy, but she ultimately chose to undergo the procedure. Chemotherapy was difficult for her, but she was thankful for her family's support. Mary underwent surgery after completing her therapy, and she has been cancer-free for five years.

Case Study 2: Radiation Therapy: After receiving a stage 2 colon cancer diagnosis, radiation therapy and surgery were advised for John. John was originally apprehensive about radiation therapy because he was worried that it may harm healthy tissue. However, he chose to go with radiation therapy after consulting with his medical staff and hearing from others who had received the treatment. With the assistance of his medical team, John was able to control the side effects, which included moderate weariness and skin irritation. John underwent surgery and has been cancer-free for three years after finishing radiation therapy.

Case Study 3: Surgery Susan was found to have stage 1 colon cancer, and surgery was advised. Susan was originally apprehensive about having surgery because she was worried about possible hazards and the length of the recovery process. However, she made the decision to have surgery after speaking with her medical team and learning more about its advantages. Susan has been cancer-free for two years thanks to a successful surgery.

Tom was diagnosed with stage 4 colon cancer and given the advice to get chemotherapy and surgery. Case Study 4 - Alternative Therapies: Tom was diagnosed with stage 4 colon cancer. Tom chose to look into alternative treatments like herbal medicines and dietary changes because he was wary about conventional therapies. Tom thought that the alternative treatments improved his general health even if he did not experience a major change in his cancer.

These first-person accounts show the variety of colon cancer experiences that people have and the significance of selecting a course of treatment that is appropriate for each patient's particular circumstances. While there is no one-size-fits-all method for treating colon cancer, talking to others who have been there can offer insightful advice and motivation to those who are dealing with a cancer diagnosis. To make an informed decision regarding their course of treatment and to put their general wellbeing first throughout the process, people should consult carefully with their medical team and loved ones.

CHAPTER TWO

Side Effects: Coping with Treatment Challenges

An essential part of controlling colon cancer is being aware of the usual adverse effects of treatment. Although the adverse effects of each treatment choice may vary, it is vital to be aware of them so that you can take the necessary action to manage them. Common negative effects of colon cancer treatment include:

Chemotherapy - Using medications to kill cancer cells, chemotherapy is a frequent treatment for colon cancer. Chemotherapy side effects might include diarrhoea, vomiting, exhaustion, hair loss, mouth sores, and a higher risk of infection.

Another treatment option is radiation therapy, which employs high-energy radiation to kill cancer cells. Fatigue, skin irritability, and diarrhea can be side effects of radiation therapy.

Surgery - Surgery is frequently used to remove colon malignant tissue. The aftereffects of surgery can include discomfort, exhaustion, and gastrointestinal problems.

Targeted therapy is a form of treatment in which medications are used to specifically target proteins or genes that play a role in the development of cancer cells. Targeted therapy may cause skin rashes, nausea, vomiting, or diarrhea as side effects.

Immunotherapy is a form of treatment that makes use of the immune system to combat cancer. Immunotherapy's adverse effects can include fatigue, fever, and muscle aches.

Although managing these side effects might be difficult, there are steps people can take to do so.

Some methods for coping with adverse effects include:

Maintaining hydration - Getting enough fluids can help to control side symptoms including diarrhea and nausea.

Eating a balanced diet might help control side effects like exhaustion and keep your health overall when you're receiving treatment.

Getting enough sleep is crucial for managing side effects like exhaustion throughout treatment.

In order for your medical staff to properly assist you in managing any adverse effects you have, it is crucial that you communicate them to them.

Seeking assistance from family and friends - Having a support network throughout treatment can be beneficial in assisting with the mental and physical issues associated with cancer therapy.

People with colon cancer can preserve their quality of life while receiving treatment by being aware of the usual side effects and taking the necessary precautions to control them. To control side effects and put their general wellbeing first while undergoing treatment, patients must collaborate closely with their medical team.

Tips for managing physical symptoms (nausea, fatigue, etc.)

Physical side effects from cancer treatment might include pain, exhaustion, and nausea. Managing these symptoms might be difficult, but there are things people can do to make them go away. For controlling physical side effects when receiving cancer therapy, consider the following:

Vomiting and nausea - Vomiting and nausea are frequent side effects of chemotherapy and radiation treatment. Try eating small, frequent meals throughout the day, staying away from strong scents or flavors, and sipping on clear liquids like water or ginger tea to control these symptoms. Your doctor may also recommend anti-nausea medicine to treat these symptoms.

Fatigue is a typical side effect of cancer therapy that can make it challenging to carry on with daily activities. Try to conserve your energy during the day by taking frequent pauses, giving the most critical tasks the highest priority, and obtaining adequate sleep to manage weariness. Walking or yoga are two gentle exercises that can assist increase energy and enhance general wellbeing.

Pain is a frequent sign of cancer and may be brought on by the disease itself or a side effect of treatment. Consult your doctor about pain-reduction measures including prescription drugs, physical therapy, or alternative treatments like acupuncture or massage.

Mouth sores - Mouth sores can be brought on by chemotherapy or radiation treatment and can be uncomfortable for both speaking and eating. Avoid foods that are hot, spicy, or acidic, and try to consume soft foods to manage mouth sores.

Using a specific mouthwash or rinsing your mouth with saltwater can also aid in pain relief and healing.

Constipation - Constipation is a typical adverse effect of painkillers and can be made worse by inactivity. Try eating a high-fiber diet, drinking plenty of water, and doing light activity like walking to treat constipation. Stool softeners that are available only by prescription or over-the-counter can also aid in managing constipation.

The side effects of chemotherapy and radiation therapy may include diarrhea. Eat modest, frequent meals throughout the day and stay away from items like high-fat or greasy foods that might make diarrhea symptoms worse. Loperamide and other over-the-counter drugs can also help to reduce symptoms.

Any physical symptoms should be discussed with your doctor.

Any physical symptoms must be discussed with your medical team in order for them to provide you with effective management. During treatment, cancer patients can assist to maintain their quality of life by being proactive in managing their physical symptoms.

Coping with emotional and mental health challenges

The emotional and mental health of an individual can be significantly impacted by cancer. It can be difficult to deal with the emotional and mental health difficulties that come with a cancer diagnosis, but there are methods that can be useful.

Seeking support - Talking with family, friends, or support groups through trying times might help you feel better emotionally. Support groups offer a sense of belonging and connection, enabling people to talk with others who are going through similar things.

Counseling - Talking about one's emotional and mental health issues in a safe environment with a qualified therapist can help people. Therapy can assist patients in overcoming emotional difficulties that may emerge during cancer treatment, such as anxiety, depression, and other mental health issues.

Mindfulness - Meditation, yoga, and deep breathing exercises are mindfulness techniques that can assist people in controlling their stress and anxiety. During the course of treatment or recovery, these techniques might be extremely beneficial.

Self-care - Self-care activities, such as making time for hobbies or exercising, can provide patients a sense of normalcy and control while they are receiving treatment. During this trying period, it's crucial to look after one's physical and emotional well-being.

Medication - In some situations, using medication to treat depression or anxiety symptoms may be necessary. It is crucial to talk to your healthcare professional about any mental health issues so they can advise you on your treatment options.

Spiritual activities - Taking part in spiritual activities, such as prayer or meditation, can assist people in discovering a sense of meaning and purpose through trying times. In times of ambiguity, spiritual practices can offer consolation and encouragement.

It's critical to keep in mind that finding coping mechanisms that are effective for you takes time and is a process while dealing with emotional and mental health difficulties. There is no shame in asking for assistance when you need it, so do so whenever you need to. Cancer patients can help to maintain their quality of life and well-being by taking proactive measures to manage their emotional and mental health difficulties.

CHAPTER THREE

Support Systems: Finding Help Along the Way

B uilding a support network is crucial for those receiving treatment for cancer because receiving a diagnosis can be emotionally and physically taxing. Throughout the cancer journey, support networks can offer emotional, practical, and physical support.

Here are some justifications on why creating a support system is crucial:

Support network - Receiving a cancer diagnosis may be a lonely and isolating experience. Having a support network can help. Speaking with friends or family members might make you feel connected and at ease. A network of others going through comparable situations can be found through support groups.

Support network members can offer practical assistance with

daily tasks like cooking, cleaning, and running errands. Cancer treatment can be physically taxing. By reducing some of the stress associated with therapy, practical support enables people to concentrate on their health and wellbeing.

Medical support - Creating a network of friends and family members that includes medical experts can give you access to resources and medical assistance. Doctors, nurses, and social workers can all be a part of a medical support network and offer direction and encouragement while undergoing treatment.

Advocacy - Having a support system during therapy can offer advocacy. Support groups can assist people in interacting with healthcare professionals, navigating the healthcare system, and selecting the best course of therapy.

Creating a network of supporters can give one a sense of belonging and community. Finding others who are experiencing similar things as you might give you a sense of mutual understanding and support. Reaching out to friends and family, signing up for a support group, making connections with medical experts, and looking for assistance from other sources like online communities can all be part of building a support network. It's crucial to keep in mind that creating a support system is a process, and finding the correct resources could take some time. People with cancer might feel less alone and more supported during their cancer journey by creating a support network.

Finding community resources for cancer patients and survivors

Discovering local resources can be a great help to cancer patients and survivors. Here are some methods for locating neighborhood resources:

Cancer groups - There are a large number of cancer organizations that provide assistance, information, and advocacy for patients and survivors. These groups offer a variety of services, including support groups, educational initiatives, financial aid, and transportation options. The American Cancer Society, CancerCare, and the Leukemia & Lymphoma Society are a few examples of cancer organizations.

Support groups - For those with cancer, support groups can foster a sense of belonging and community. Local hospitals and community centers often provide support groups, as do numerous cancer organizations. People who might not have access to offline support groups can benefit from online support groups as well.

Social workers - Social workers can offer cancer patients helpful resources and assistance. Social workers can offer emotional support, connect people with local resources, and assist people with navigating the healthcare system. Social workers who can offer these services are employed by many hospitals and cancer treatment facilities.

Community centers - A lot of community centers provide

resources and programs for cancer patients and survivors, including support groups, exercise classes, and nutrition courses. Local libraries might also have resources and knowledge about community cancer support services.

Online resources - There are a variety of online tools accessible for cancer patients and survivors, such as forums, support groups, and instructional materials. The American Cancer Society, Cancer.Net, and the National Comprehensive Cancer Network are a few instances of online resources.

It's crucial to keep in mind that locating community services is a process, and discovering the ones that are effective for you may take some time. People with cancer can find vital tools and assistance to help them through their cancer experience by looking for them in their local community.

Personal stories of individuals who found support in unexpected places

Some people find support in unexpected places, despite the fact that friends, family, and medical professionals' support is crucial for cancer patients and survivors. Here are some first-person accounts of people who discovered encouragement in unlikely places:

An onboard stranger - After receiving a breast cancer diagnosis, one woman sought comfort from an onboard stranger. The stranger, a fellow passenger, started talking to the woman while she was her route to her chemotherapy appointment. The stranger, who had previously endured cancer, gave the woman advice and comfort. The woman later posted her experience on social media, where it quickly gained popularity and motivated others to do the same.

A hairstylist - Hair loss is a typical side effect of cancer therapy, and some people find support from hairstylists who focus on helping cancer patients. One breast cancer survivor talked about how she found a hairstylist who gave her confidence while she was through treatment. The hairstylist made the woman feel confident despite losing her hair by creating a welcoming and encouraging environment.

A pet - For those with cancer, pets can offer company and emotional support. A cancer patient found solace in his cat, who would cuddle up next to him during chemotherapy. During a stressful moment, the cat brought me solace and a sense of serenity.

A hobby - Having a pastime can give you a feeling of purpose during cancer treatment and can also serve as a distraction. One breast cancer patient found comfort in crocheting. During therapy, knitting gave me a creative outlet and a sense of accomplishment. Additionally, she joined a knitting group where she discovered a group of receptive people who enjoyed the same pastime.

Finding support in a spiritual group might be beneficial for some people going through cancer treatment. One ovarian cancer patient sought assistance from her church family. She participated in prayer meetings, went to church services, and got assistance from other churchgoers.

Finding help in unexpected locations might serve as a reminder that help can come in many different forms, therefore it is crucial to keep an open mind.

CHAPTER FOUR

Life After Cancer: Adjusting to a New Normal

Cancer survivorship can be a difficult and trying period. It might be challenging to cope with potential physical and mental changes, but there are services and coping mechanisms available. Here are some suggestions for managing the physical and psychological adjustments of survivorship:

Address physical changes - Addressing bodily changes is important since survivors may go through physical changes like lymphedema, exhaustion, and pain. Any physical changes should be discussed with a healthcare professional so that a management strategy may be created. This could involve adjustments to one's lifestyle, medicine, or physical treatment.

Manage emotional changes - Being a survivor can result in a variety of emotions, including worry, despair, and recurrence fear. Seeking out help from family, friends, mental health specialists, or support groups is crucial. Emotional shifts can be managed with the aid of relaxation practices like yoga, meditation, and others.

Self-care: Self-care is crucial for general health and wellbeing, therefore practice it. This could involve getting some exercise, eating well, and sleeping sufficiently. Participating in enjoyable activities can enhance mood and general well-being.

Deal with relationships – The cancer experience may have an impact on relationships, and survivors may need to deal with changes in relationships with loved ones. Any issue must be addressed via communication, and getting support from a therapist or counselor can be helpful.

Discuss sexuality and intimacy. Cancer and its treatment may have an impact on these areas. It is crucial to discuss any worries with a healthcare professional and, if necessary, get support from a therapist or counselor.

Join a group of supporters- Cancer survivorship support groups can foster a sense of belonging and comprehension. Making connections with people who have gone through similar things and exchanging coping mechanisms for survivorship can be beneficial.

Every person's road toward cancer survival is different. Although adjusting to physical and emotional changes can be challenging, survivors can go through this new stage of their lives with resiliency and strength with the help of support and self-care.

Navigating the fear of recurrence

For many cancer survivors, the fear of a relapse is a common and natural worry. Although overcoming this anxiety can be difficult, there are techniques that can be useful. Here are some suggestions for overcoming the fear of repetition:

Speak with a healthcare professional – It is crucial to discuss any recurrence-related worries with a healthcare professional. They can offer details on the possibility of a recurrence and any possible prevention actions.

Create a survivorship plan: A survivorship plan can serve as a guide for managing continuing medical requirements and can help reduce recurrence concern. This schedule could include examinations, exams, and screenings.

Don't worry about the future; instead, keep your attention on the here and now. Yoga and meditation are both mindfulness practices that can assist with maintaining present-moment awareness.

Address emotional issues: Anxiety and depression among other emotions might be triggered by the fear of a repeat occurrence. It's crucial to deal with emotional issues by getting help from family members or mental health experts.

Exercise, eating well, and getting enough sleep are examples of healthy practices that can enhance general wellbeing and lower the likelihood of recurrence.

Join an advocacy group - Making connections with other

cancer survivors who share your worries might help you feel understood and connected. assistance groups can teach coping mechanisms for dealing with recurrence anxiety and offer a safe haven for emotional assistance. Although navigating the fear of recurrence can be difficult, it is possible to manage this worry and go on with resilience and strength with the correct support and tactics.

Strategies for living a healthy and fulfilling life after cancer

Many cancer patients who have completed treatment aim to lead healthy, rewarding lives. This can entail adapting a healthy lifestyle, coping with emotional and physical difficulties, and discovering a new sense of purpose. Following cancer, these are some tips for leading a healthy and happy life:

Make self-care a priority - Emotional and physical well-being depend on self-care. This might entail stress management techniques, a good diet, frequent exercise, and sleeping enough hours.

Participate in joyful pursuits - Achieving happiness and contentment in life is crucial for overall health. This may be engaging in hobbies, spending time with close friends and family, or giving back to a worthwhile cause.

Address emotional and menatal health needs - Cancer survivors may struggle with emotional and mental health issues including despair or anxiety. To overcome these difficulties, seek assistance from support groups or mental health specialists.

Keep a positive view - Keeping a positive outlook can enhance general wellbeing and assist in overcoming any obstacles. This could entail being grateful, emphasizing your abilities and successes, and looking for supportive connections.

Use mindfulness practices to reduce stress and anxiety and to improve your general wellbeing. Examples of these techniques are yoga or meditation.

Get in touch with other cancer survivors – Having a sense of community and understanding might come through getting in touch with other cancer survivors. Support groups or online discussion boards can offer emotional support and coping mechanisms for survivorship.

Look for fresh chances - After therapy, cancer patients could discover a new sense of purpose. This could entail exploring new career prospects, going on vacation, or finding a new interest or hobby.

Living a healthy and full life after cancer can be difficult, but it is possible to do so with resiliency and strength if you have the correct strategies and support. Cancer survivors can thrive in their new stage of life by putting self-care first, discovering joy and purpose, and getting help when they need it.

6

CHAPTER FIVE

The Power of Advocacy: Making a Difference

In the healthcare system, speaking up for oneself and others is a crucial part of cancer survivorship. It entails actively participating in your own care, successfully communicating with healthcare professionals, and speaking up for the needs of other patients. Here are some tips for using the healthcare system to advocate for you and other people:

Learn about your condition and available treatments so that you may make an educated choice about your care. This can entail looking up information about your disease online or talking to medical professionals.

Effective communication with healthcare professionals is essential if you want to receive the treatment you require. This may entail posing inquiries, voicing worries, and offering feedback regarding your care.

Maintaining a record of your medical information will assist guarantee that all healthcare professionals have access to crucial data on your treatment.

Getting second opinions from different healthcare professionals can give you more information and assist you in making decisions about your care that are more informed.

Speak up when something isn't working or when you need more support. This is what it means to be an advocate for your needs. In order to do this, you might need to ask for more tests, prescription drugs, or referrals to different medical specialists.

Advocacy for the needs of others entails speaking up on behalf of other patients who may not be able to speak up for themselves. Raising awareness about problems like patient safety, healthcare inequities, or access to care may be necessary for this.

Participate in advocacy organizations - Participating in advocacy organizations can provide you a platform to encourage change in the healthcare system and raise awareness of critical concerns.

It might be difficult to speak up for oneself and others in the healthcare system, but doing so is crucial to raising patient safety and treatment quality. You may have a positive impact on the healthcare system and encourage improved results for all patients by educating yourself, communicating clearly with healthcare professionals, and advocating for your needs as well as the needs of others.

The importance of cancer research and fundraising

In order to better understand cancer and provide novel therapies and technologies to enhance patient outcomes, cancer research is essential. Raising money for cancer research is crucial to advancing important research and offering hope to cancer patients and their families.

Here are several justifications for the significance of cancer research and fundraising:

Advancing scientific understanding - Cancer research contributes to improvements in our knowledge of the biology, risk factors, prevention, and treatment of cancer. We can create novel medicines, enhance current ones, and find new targets for intervention by conducting research.

Enhancing patient outcomes - New treatments that have improved patient outcomes and survival rates have been developed as a result of cancer research. To name a few, these improvements include those made in chemotherapy, radiation therapy, targeted medicines, and immunotherapy.

Lessening the impact of cancer - Advances in early detection and prevention made possible by cancer research have the potential to lessen the impact of cancer on people, families, and society at large.

Supporting patients and families – Support for cancer patients and families affected by the disease is provided by fundraising efforts for cancer research. This covers funding for efforts promoting survivorship, patient support services, and access to care for underserved groups.

Driving innovation and teamwork - The study of cancer brings together professionals from diverse sectors to work together and provide creative answers to challenging issues. This includes professionals who collaborate to enhance the science of cancer research, such as researchers, doctors, patient advocates, and others.

Increasing awareness and education - Raising money for cancer research aids in spreading knowledge and understanding of cancer, its effects on people and families, and the value of early identification and prevention.

In conclusion, funding for cancer research and development is crucial for expanding our knowledge of the disease and creating novel therapies and technology to enhance patient outcomes. We can try to lessen the impact of cancer and offer hope to those impacted by the disease by supporting cancer research and fundraising initiatives.

Personal stories of individuals who have become advocates for colon cancer awareness and prevention.

Survivors of colon cancer and those who care about them frequently become ardent supporters of colon cancer education and prevention, trying to increase public awareness, encourage screening, and aid in research activities. Here are some first-person accounts of some people who have become colon cancer prevention and awareness activists:

Journalist Katie Couric has been a strong proponent of colon cancer awareness and prevention since her spouse passed away from the disease. To encourage others to get examined, she had a colonoscopy on live television. She also started the National Colorectal Cancer Research Alliance to fund research and awareness programs.

Eric Stonestreet: After learning that his mother had colon cancer, the Modern Family actor started to promote colon cancer screenings. He has collaborated with the American Cancer Society to promote awareness of the value of early detection and screening.

Stacy Hurt: After receiving a stage 4 colon cancer diagnosis at the age of 44, Stacy Hurt turned into a patient advocate and motivational speaker, using her experience to spread awareness of the disease and inspire others to be screened. She is also a member of the Colon Cancer Coalition's board of directors.

Andrew Albert: Andrew Albert established the charity group

"No Butts About It" to spread the word about the value of screening and early detection after losing his father to colon cancer. Colonoscopies are being given away without charge to those in need thanks to a collaboration between the organization and local charities and healthcare providers.

Robert Marsilje: Tom Marsilje, a cancer researcher and patient advocate, was 45 years old when he received his stage 4 colon cancer diagnosis. In addition to working with the Colorectal Cancer Alliance and other groups to advance research and awareness programs, he has developed into a strong supporter of patient access to clinical trials.

These are just a handful of the numerous people who have taken the lead in raising awareness of and preventing colon cancer. They are aiming to improve colon cancer patient outcomes and increase awareness of the value of screening and early diagnosis through their personal experiences and advocacy activities.